THE ENDOMORPH DIET COOKBOOK FOR BEGINNERS (SENIORS)

NATALIE BROWN

Copyright ©2024.

TABLE OF CONTENTS

WHAT IS AN ENDOMORPH?

An endomorph is one of the three main body types, or somatotypes, as defined by the body type diet. Although this word often has a negative connotation, it can be used as a neutral term because it's natural for some people to have larger or thicker bodies.

The Other Body Types

The other two types are ectomorph and mesomorph. **Ectomorphs** tend to be thin and have long, lanky limbs. **Mesomorphs**, meanwhile, are more muscular and have hourglass-shaped bodies, past research shows.

How the Body Type Diet Works and How to Know if You're an Endomorph

Endomorphs are primarily characterized by their propensity to store fat, as well as a wider waistline and bigger bone structure, according to the book Integrative Approaches for Health. Catudal says that endomorphs tend to gain weight more easily compared with ectomorphs and mesomorphs. Even when eating a similar diet as another body type, an endomorph will tend to hold on to more excess fat, he says.

In addition, this excess fat often deposits around the waist.

FOOD LIST FOR AN ENDOMORPH

The thinking goes that endomorphs do best when they focus on reducing calorie intake and taking in more protein, healthy fats, and low-carb foods. Catudal says this approach will help them trim fat, reduce their waistline, and improve insulin resistance. Here are the foods you're allowed to eat on an endomorph diet.

Meat and Fish

- Chicken
- Turkey
- Salmon
- Cod

Dairy

- Yogurt
- Milk

Fruit and vegetables

- Berries
- Apples

- Pears
- Asparagus
- Zucchini
- Tomatoes
- Onions
- Greens (spinach, kale, romaine)

Nuts and seeds

- Nut and seed butter
- Almonds
- Pistachios
- Sunflower seeds
- Pumpkin seeds

GRAINS AND STARCHY VEGETABLES

- Sweet potatoes
- Squash
- Quinoa
- Brown rice
- Beans
- Oats

ENDOMORPH DIET RECIPES

LOW-CARB BACON CHEESEBURGER CASSEROLE

INGREDIENTS

- 6 ounces bacon
- 1 tablespoon avocado oil
- 1.5 pounds ground beef
- 1 teaspoon onion powder
- 1 teaspoon parsley
- 1 teaspoon garlic powder
- 1 teaspoon salt
- ½ teaspoon pepper
- 20 ounces frozen cauliflower rice (see notes above for fresh cauliflower)
- ⅓ cup coconut flour 40 grams
- ¼ teaspoon salt
- Sauce
- 1 tablespoon butter
- 1 tablespoon coconut flour
- 1 ½ cups heavy cream
- 2 tablespoons mustard
- 8 ounces cheddar cheese

INSTRUCTIONS

1. Place ½ cup of the sauce on the bottom of a 9 by 13 baking dish.
2. Spread the cauliflower mixture on top of the sauce as evenly as possible.
3. Place 4 ounces of cheddar over the cauliflower rice.
4. Spread the ground beef over the cheddar evenly.
5. Pour half of the remaining sauce over the beef.
6. Place the remaining cheddar over the sauce.
7. Pour the remaining sauce over the top and sprinkle with chopped bacon.
8. Cover and bake 30 minutes.
9. Uncover and bake an additional 5 minutes.
10. Allow to cool out of the oven for 15-20 minutes before slicing and serving.

BIG MAC SALAD (LOW CARB, GLUTEN-FREE)

INGREDIENTS

SALAD

- 1 lb Ground beef
- 1 tsp Sea salt
- 1/4 tsp Black pepper
- 8 oz Romaine lettuce (or iceberg if desired)
- 1 cup Tomatoes (chopped)
- 3/4 cup Cheddar cheese (shredded)
- 1/2 cup Pickles (diced)
- DRESSING
- 1/2 cup Mayonnaise
- 2 tbsp Pickles (diced)
- 2 tsp Mustard
- 1 tsp White vinegar
- 1/2 tsp Smoked paprika
- 1 1/2 tbsp Besti Powdered Erythritol (or any sweetener of choice; adjust to taste)

INSTRUCTIONS

1. Cook ground beef in a skillet over high heat. Season with sea salt and black pepper. Stir fry, breaking up the pieces with a spatula, for about 7-10 minutes, until the beef is browned and moisture has evaporated.
2. Meanwhile, puree all the dressing ingredients in a blender. If dressing is thicker than you like, thin out with water or oil and puree again. Adjust sweetener to taste. Refrigerate until ready to serve.
3. Combine the remaining salad ingredients in a large bowl. Add the ground beef. Toss with dressing.

MONGOLIAN BEEF SATAY

INGREDIENTS

- 2 1/2 lbs sirloin steaks
- chopped peanuts for garnish
- wood skewers

Marinade:

- 2 Tbsp. peanut oil or veg. oil if you are allergic
- 1 tsp. ginger
- 1 Tbsp. minced garlic
- red pepper flakes to taste
- 1/2 c. soy sauce
- 1/2 c. dark brown sugar

Spicy Dipping Sauce:

- 1/2 c. mayonnaise
- 1/4 c. sour cream
- 1 tsp. sriracha hot sauce

- 1 tsp. lime juice
- 1/2 tsp garlic powder

INSTRUCTIONS

1. Mix together the marinade ingredients in a large bowl.
2. Cut the beef into long thin strips, then stir it into the marinade. Cover and refrigerate for at least 3 hours. About an hour before serving, mix together the sauce ingredients and refrigerate. Then soak the wood skewers in a water bath. (This will keep them from catching on fire during grilling).
3. About 20 minutes before serving, thread the meat onto the skewers, baste the meat with some of the marinade, then discard the excess.
4. Grill for about 6 to 7 minutes on each side over direct high heat, only turning once.
5. Garnish with chopped peanuts and serve with spicy dipping sauce.

GRILLED SHRIMP WITH ROASTED GARLIC HERB SAUCE

INGREDIENTS

- 1.5 lb uncooked large shrimp, peeled and deveined
- kosher salt and black pepper
- Extra virgin olive oil

For the Sauce:

- 1 small head garlic. top trimmed off
- 1 cup chopped fresh cilantro leaves, or basil if you can't use cilantro
- 1 lime, juice of
- 1 tablespoon dry white wine
- 3 to 4 tablespoon Extra virgin olive oil
- 2 tablespoon chili paste, or harissa paste

INSTRUCTIONS

1. Preheat your oven to 400 degrees F.

2. Roast the garlic: Trim the top off the garlic head to expose a bit of the cloves, but keep the garlic cloves intact. Drizzle generously with olive oil and wrap in foil. Roast the garlic in the heated oven for about 10 minutes or until slightly tender and fragrant. When ready, remove from the oven. Let cool briefly. then peel and crush or chop the roasted garlic as finely as possible. (See cook's tip #1)

3. Prepare the sauce: In a small bowl, combine the roasted garlic with the remaining sauce ingredients of fresh cilantro (or basil if you can't have cilantro), lime juice, white wine, extra virgin olive oil and chili paste (harissa is also an excellent option here). Whisk together and set aside.

4. Grill the shrimp: Heat an outdoor grill or an indoor griddle or cast iron skillet over high heat. Pat shrimp dry and season with salt and pepper, drizzle a little extra virgin olive oil and toss. Arrange shrimp on heated surface and cook for about 2 on one side or until the shrimp turns just pink, then flip over and cook until the shrimp turns just

pink, maybe another 1 to 2 minutes (even the largest shrimp will be ready within about 5 minutes, so be careful not to overcook it).

5. Toss the shrimp with the sauce and serve! Immediately toss the

SKINNY SLOW COOKER KUNG PAO CHICKEN

INGREDIENTS

- 1/4 tsp black pepper
- 1/8 tsp salt
- 1 - 1 1/4 lbs boneless skinless chicken breasts (about 2-3 pieces), cut into bite-sized chunks
- 3-4 tablespoons olive oil
- 4 - 6 dried red chili peppers to taste
- 2/3 cup roasted cashews or roasted peanuts
- 1 red bell pepper chopped into bite-sized pieces
- 1 medium zucchini chopped into halves

Sauce (Feel free to double the sauce if you like more sauce)

- 1/2 cup low-sodium soy sauce

- 1/2 cup water
- 3 Tablespoons honey
- 2 Tablespoons hoisin sauce
- 3 cloves garlic minced
- 1 tsp grated fresh ginger
- ¼ - 1/2 teaspoon dried red pepper chili flakes

Cornstarch slurry

- 2 Tablespoons cornstarch or arrowroot powder
- 2-3 Tablespoons water plus more as needed to thin out consistency of sauce

INSTRUCTIONS

1. In a large zip-top bag, toss in chicken, salt and black pepper. Shake until well-coated.
2. Heat a large skillet over medium-high heat. Cook chicken about 2-3 minutes on each side, until lightly browned. **Skip this step if in a pinch and add chicken directly to the slow cooker.
3. Transfer chicken into slow cooker.

4. In a medium bowl, whisk together the soy sauce, water, honey, hoisin sauce, garlic, ginger and red pepper chili flakes and pour over chicken.

5. Cover and cook on LOW for 2.5 - 4 hours or HIGH for 1.5 - 3 hours.

6. About 30 minutes before serving, whisk together the cornstarch and water in a small bowl. Stir into the slow cooker. Add the dried red chili peppers, red bell peppers, zucchini and cashews.

7. Cover and cook on HIGH for another 20-30 minutes or until the vegetables are tender and the sauce has thickened up. (Add more water to thin out sauce to your preferred consistency).

8. Sprinkle with sesame seeds, green onions and serve over rice, quinoa or zoodles, if desired.

LOW CARB CHICKEN TACO SOUP

INGREDIENTS

- 1 tbsp vegetable oil
- 1 tbsp Minced garlic

- 1 Medium onion Chopped
- 300 grams boneless skinless chicken breast Cut in to small chunks
- ¼ cup celery Chopped
- 2 cups (heaping) cabbage Shredded
- 1 Medium red bell pepper Chopped
- 1 cup plum tomato Blanched and chopped / Canned
- ½ tbsp red chili powder
- ½ tbsp chipotle chilli powder
- 1 tbsp Roasted Cumin powder
- 2 tsp Dried Oregano
- 1 tsp Red chili flakes (optional)
- 2 cups chicken stock or Water
- Salt to taste
- ½ cup sharp cheddar cheese
- ½ cup Fresh Coriander leave for garnishing
- Lemon Wedges

INSTRUCTIONS

1. Heat oil in a pot. Add minced garlic. Saute till it starts to brown.
2. Add chopped onion. Fry till it is soft and translucent.

3. Add chopped celery, followed by chicken chunks. Fry for one minute.
4. Add shredded cabbage. Cook for 2 minutes. The cabbage will start to soften.
5. Add chopped red bell pepper. Cook for 30 seconds.
6. Add Tomatoes. Mix everything well.
7. Add all the spices. Mix everything well. Cook for 2 minutes more.
8. Add Stock. Adjust seasoning. Bring the soup to a boil(cover the pan with a lid if desired)
9. Switch off the flame. Garnish with fresh coriander leaves, lemon wedges and top it with cheese while serving.

BAKED GARLIC BROWN SUGAR CHICKEN

INGREDIENTS:

- 4 boneless skinless chicken breasts
- 4 garlic cloves, minced
- 4 tablespoons brown sugar
- 3 teaspoons olive oil

INSTRUCTIONS:

1. Preheat oven to 500°F and lightly grease a casserole dish.
2. In small sauté pan, sauté garlic with the oil until tender.
3. Remove from heat and stir in brown sugar.
4. Place chicken breasts in a prepared baking dish and cover with the garlic and brown sugar mixture.
5. Add salt and pepper to taste.
6. Bake uncovered for 15-30 minutes.

BAKED CHICKEN FAJITA ROLL-UPS

INGREDIENTS

For the Marinade:

- 2 Tbsp olive oil
- Juice of half a lime
- 1 clove garlic, minced
- 1 tsp. chili powder
- ½ tsp. cumin
- ½ tsp. dried oregano
- ½ tsp. salt
- Pinch of cayenne pepper (optional)
- 2 Tbsp cilantro, chopped

For the Chicken:

- 3 chicken breasts or 6 thin sliced chicken cutlets ¼-inch thick
- ½ red bell pepper, sliced
- ½ yellow bell pepper, sliced
- ½ green bell pepper, sliced

INSTRUCTIONS

1. In a small bowl, whisk together olive oil, lime juice, garlic, chili powder, cumin, oregano, salt, cayenne (if using) and cilantro. Set aside.
2. For the chicken breasts, if you purchased pre-sliced chicken cutlets then skip to the next step. If using chicken breasts, slice them longways into 2 even slices and firmly pound the chicken using the smooth side of a meat tenderizer to an even thickness of about ¼ inch.
3. Place chicken cutlets into a large resealable freezer bag and pour marinade over top, making sure they are completely coated. Allow chicken to marinate for a minimum of one hour to overnight.

4. Once chicken has marinated, evenly place 6 bell pepper slices in the middle of the chicken cutlet, roll up and secure with a toothpick. Repeat this step until all the cutlets have been rolled up and place seam side down in a prepared baking dish.
5. Brush tops of chicken with remaining marinade and bake, uncovered, at 375 for about 25 to 30 minutes or until the juices run clear. Serve and enjoy!

LOW CARB CLOUD BREAD RECIPE MADE WITH BAKING SODA

INGREDIENTS

- 3 eggs separated
- 3 Tablespoons cream cheese
- 1/4 teaspoon baking powder or cream of tarter
- Optional: 1/2 teaspoon Rosemary seasoning
- Optional: 1/2 teaspoon sea salt
- Optional: 1/4 teaspoon pepper

INSTRUCTIONS

1. Preheat the oven to 350 degrees Fahrenheit

2. Separate the egg yolks from the egg whites.
3. In the egg yolks bowl, add the cream cheese and mix it with a hand mixer until it's fully blended.
4. In the egg whites bowl, add the baking powder and mix it with a hand mixer until the egg whites are fluffy and form peaks that hold their shape (as seen in the photos below). This process will take the longest at about 5 minutes or so.
5. Next, you will combine both bowls together into one. Fold the mixtures together until the are fully mixed but don't over mix these ingredients. It's important to keep the egg whites nice and fluffy. Over mixing these ingredients will cause a thick liquidy mixture and that won't work for this bread recipe. There will be no way to correct this recipe if you over mix it. You will want to do this rather quickly so the ingredients don't melt back to a liquid consistency.
6. Spray the baking pan with a non-stick cooking spray and drop small spoonfuls of the batter onto a cookie sheet with a bakers mat to prevent sticking. Use the spoon to

spread out the batter in the size of bread you want. Now sprinkle any seasonings you want on the top of each bread patty.

7. I made hamburger bun sized bread patties. I am able to get between 10 and 12 slices of bread out of this recipe.

8. Bake it for about 15 to 20 minutes. My oven tends to cook at a higher temperature so I know my recipes get done faster. Usually, 15 minutes is all it takes for me. Be sure to watch it when it's close to the 15-minute mark. They should be a light golden brown color when they are done.

CREAMY GARLIC BUTTER TUSCAN SHRIMP

INGREDIENTS

- 2 tablespoons salted butter
- 6 cloves garlic, finely diced
- 1 pound (500 g) shrimp (or prawns), tails on or off
- 1 small yellow onion, diced
- 1/2 cup white wine (OPTIONAL)

- 5 oz (150 g) jarred sun dried tomato strips in oil, drained (reserve 1 teaspoon of the jarred oil for cooking)
- 1 3/4 cups half and half SEE NOTES
- Salt and pepper, to taste
- 3 cups baby spinach leaves, washed
- 2/3 cup fresh grated Parmesan cheese
- 1 teaspoon cornstarch (cornflour) mixed with 1 tablespoons of water (optional)***
- 2 teaspoons dried Italian herbs
- 1 tablespoon fresh parsley, chopped

INSTRUCTIONS

1. Heat a large skillet over medium-high heat. Melt the butter and add in the garlic and fry until fragrant (about one minute). Add in the shrimp and fry two minutes on each side, until just cooked through and pink. Transfer to a bowl; set aside.
2. Fry the onion in the butter remaining in the skillet. Pour in the white wine (if using), and allow to reduce to half, while scraping any bits off of the bottom of the pan. Add the sun dried tomatoes and fry for 1-2 minutes to release their flavours.

3. Reduce heat to low-medium heat, add the half and half and bring to a gentle simmer, while stirring occasionally. Season with salt and pepper to your taste.

4. Add in the spinach leaves and allow to wilt in the sauce, and add in the parmesan cheese. Allow sauce to simmer for a further minute until cheese melts through the sauce. (For a thicker sauce, add the milk/cornstarch mixture to the centre of the pan, and continue to simmer while quickly stirring the mixture through until the sauce thickens.)

5. Add the shrimp back into the pan; sprinkle with the herbs and parsley, and stir through.

6. Serve over pasta, rice or steamed veg.

EASY ASIAN STEAK BITES

INGREDIENTS

- 1 and 1/2 pounds flank steak sirloin steak also works
- 4 tablespoons Kikkoman Less Sodium Soy Sauce
- 2 tablespoons honey

- 1 tablespoon Kikkoman Thai Style Chili Sauce
- 2 tablespoons + 1/2 teaspoon sesame oil separated
- 1 tablespoon minced garlic
- Optional: toasted sesame seeds

Dipping Sauce

- Scant 1/2 cup real mayo
- 2 large limes
- 3 teaspoons Kikkoman Sriracha Hot Chili Sauce
- 1 teaspoon white sugar

INSTRUCTIONS

1. Cut the steak: Trim excess fat from the meat and then cut strips of the meat against the grain and just barely less than 1 inch wide.
2. Rotate the strips and cut into bite-sized pieces. (Remove any large chunks of fat or gristle.)

3. In a large bowl, whisk together the soy sauce, honey, chili paste, 1/2 teaspoon sesame oil, and garlic.

4. Place the cut meat pieces into the mixture and toss well to coat. Cover tightly and marinate for at least 20 minutes and up to 4 hours.

5. (While it is marinating, whip together the sauce!)

6. When ready to cook, turn on your ventilation fan.

7. Heat a large nonstick skillet over medium-high to high heat. As the pan heats, add in 1 tablespoon of sesame oil.

8. Place some of the steak in the pan in a single layer. It should sizzle loudly AS SOON as it hits the pan to get a nice sear. (If it doesn't, the pan isn't hot enough.)

9. Don't stir or move the meat for 30 to 45 seconds. You want it to sizzle and brown on one side. Quickly flip the bites over and cook for an additional 30 to 45 seconds-just long enough to sear the outside of the meat but not cook the inside. You want these bites tender so avoid over-cooking.

10. Remove all of the cooked steak bites to a plate. Add the remaining sesame oil to the pan and repeat the cooking process with the next batch just as before.
11. Once all the meat is cooked, topped with sesame seeds if desired and enjoy with the dipping sauce.

Dipping Sauce

1. Zest part of 1 lime to get 1/2 teaspoon lime zest and then juice 2 limes to get about 3-4 tablespoons lime juice.
2. Combine the mayo, lime juice, lime zest, Sriracha, and white sugar in a bowl. Add some salt + pepper to taste. Stir well and then taste (add additional lime or Sriracha to personal preference).

CRISPY PARMESAN GARLIC CHICKEN WITH ZUCCHINI

INGREDIENTS

- 2 Chicken Breasts sliced in half, or 4 thin chicken breasts
- 8 Tablespoons butter divided
- ½ cup Italian Bread Crumbs
- ½ cup plus 1 Tablespoon grated parmesan divided
- ¼ cup flour
- 2 medium zucchini sliced
- 2 garlic cloves minced

INSTRUCTIONS

1. In a large skillet over medium heat melt 2 Tablespoons butter. To make the chicken: Melt the remaining 4 tablespoons of butter in a shallow dish. In another shallow dish combine bread crumbs, parmesan cheese, and flour. Dip the chicken in the butter and then coat in the bread crumb mixture and place in skillet.
2. Cook on each side for about 3-4 minutes until the outside is crispy and the chicken is cooked throughout. Set aside on plate.

3. Add 2 Tablespoons of butter back to the skillet and saute the minced garlic for a minute. Add the zucchini to the skillet and saute until tender. Salt and pepper to taste and add 1 Tablespoon parmesan. Add the chicken back to the skillet and heat for a minute or so. Serve immediately.

GRILLED ASIAN GARLIC STEAK SKEWERS

INGREDIENTS

- 1 1/2 pounds top sirloin steak
- 2/3 cup soy sauce
- 6 garlic cloves minced
- 1/4 cup sesame oil
- 1/4 cup olive oil
- ½ cup sugar
- 1 Tablespoon grated ginger

- 2 tbsp sesame seeds (I like using the Japanese assorted sesame seeds but any will work)
- 1 red onion cut into one inch pieces
- 1 green bell pepper cut into one inch pieces
- 1 yellow bell pepper cut into one inch pieces
- 1 red bell pepper cut into one inch pieces
- skewers
- Sliced green onions for garnish

INSTRUCTIONS

1. Cut steak into one inch cubes.
2. In a large bowl whisk together soy sauce, garlic, sesame oil, olive oil, sugar, ginger and sesame seeds. Add the steak and toss to coat in marinade. Marinate for 3 hours or overnight.
3. Preheat the grill to medium high heat. Thread the meat, red onion, and bell pepper onto the skewers. Grill for 8-10 minutes until the meat is done to desired liking.

CREAMY HERB CHICKEN

INGREDIENTS

For The Chicken:

- 4 chicken breasts (pounded 1/2-inch thin)
- 2 teaspoons each of onion powder and garlic powder
- 1 teaspoon fresh chopped parsley
- 1/2 teaspoon each of dried thyme and dried rosemary*
- salt and pepper , to season

For The Sauce:

- 4 cloves garlic , minced (or 1 tablespoon minced garlic)
- 1 teaspoon fresh chopped parsley
- 1/2 teaspoon each of dried thyme and dried rosemary
- 1 cup milk (or half and half)*
- Salt and freshly ground black pepper , to taste

- 1 teaspoon cornstarch mixed with 1 tablespoon water , until smooth

INSTRUCTIONS

1. Coat chicken breasts with the onion and garlic powders and herbs. Season generously with salt and pepper.
2. Heat 1 tablespoon of oil a large pan or skillet over medium-high heat and cook chicken breasts until opaque and no longer pink inside (about 5 minutes each side, depending on thickness). Transfer to a plate; set aside.
3. To the same pan or skillet, heat another 2 teaspoons of olive oil and sauté garlic, with parsley, thyme and rosemary, for about 1 minute, or until fragrant.
4. Stir in milk (or cream); season with salt and pepper, to taste.
5. Bring to a boil; add the cornstarch mixture to the centre of the pan, quickly stirring, until sauce has thickened slightly. Reduce heat and simmer gently for a further minute to allow the sauce to thicken more.

6. Return chicken to the skillet. Sprinkle with extra herbs if desired. Serve immediately.

CREAMY PARMESAN HERB CHICKEN MUSHROOM

INGREDIENTS

FOR THE CHICKEN:

- 6 chicken thighs (skin on or off, bone in or out)*
- 2-3 teaspoons garlic powder
- Salt and pepper

FOR THE SAUCE:

- 1 tablespoon minced garlic
- 400 g (14 oz) cups sliced mushrooms (1½ cups)
- 1 teaspoons dried basil
- 1 teaspoons dried oregano
- 2 teaspoons fresh chopped parsley
- 1½ cups evaporated milk*** (half and half or cream if using: see notes)
- 1 teaspoon chicken bullion powder (or stock powder)

- Salt and pepper to taste
- 1 tablespoon cornstarch (cornflour) mixed with 2 tablespoons of extra 2% milk****
- 3/4 cup fresh grated Parmesan cheese , divided
- 1/4 cup fresh chopped parsley (EXTRA), to serve

OPTIONAL ADD IN:

- 2 cups spinach
- 2 cups broccoli florets, lightly steamed

INSTRUCTIONS

1. Preheat oven to 200°C | 400°F.
2. Season chicken with garlic powder, salt and pepper.
3. Heat cooking oil spray in a large, non stick and oven-proof skillet over medium-high heat until hot. Sear chicken thighs until

golden and crispy on each side (about 3-4 minutes each side).

4. Transfer chicken to the oven and roast until completely cooked through, (about 25-30 minutes).

5. Once chicken is done, transfer to a warm plate and set aside. Drain some of the excess fat from the skillet, reserving 2 tablespoons for added flavour.

6. Return skillet to the stove over medium-high heat and sauté the garlic in the pan juices until fragrant (about 1 minute). Add the mushrooms, herbs and 2 teaspoons of parsley and fry until mushrooms begin to soften.

7. Reduce heat to low-medium heat, add the milk (or cream) and bring to a gentle simmer, stirring occasionally, and being careful not to boil. Add in the bullion powder and season with salt and pepper to your taste.

8. Pour the milk/cornstarch mixture to the centre of the pan, and continue to simmer while quickly stirring the mixture through until the sauce thickens.

9. Add 1/2 cup of parmesan cheese; allow sauce to simmer for a further minute until cheese melts through the sauce. Add the chicken back into the pan and allow to simmer for 1-2 minutes in the cream to take on the flavours. Taste test and add extra salt or pepper, if desired.

10. At this point, add in the optional add-ins, if desired. Allow spinach to wilt (if using).

1. Sprinkle with the remaining 1/4 cup of parsley and 1/4 cup parmesan cheese.

11. Serve with steamed rice, over steamed vegetables or pasta.

CHICKEN MARSALA

INGREDIENTS

Chicken:

- 1/2 cup all-purpose flour (plain flour)
- 1 teaspoon kosher salt
- 1 teaspoon garlic powder
- 1/2 teaspoon black cracked pepper
- 2 large boneless skinless chicken breasts, halved horizontally to make 4 fillets*
- 2 tablespoons olive oil, divided
- 4 tablespoons unsalted butter, divided

Marsala Sauce:

- 1 tablespoon unsalted butter as needed
- 8 ounces (250g) brown or Cremini mushrooms, sliced
- 4-5 cloves garlic, minced
- 3/4 cup dry Marsala wine
- 1 1/4 cup low-sodium chicken broth (or stock)
- 3/4 cup heavy cream (thickened cream, evaporated milk or half and half may also be used)**

- 2 tablespoons fresh chopped parsley

INSTRUCTIONS

1. Mix the flour, salt, garlic powder and pepper in a shallow bowl. Dredge the chicken in the flour mixture and shake off excess.
2. Heat 1 tablespoon oil and 2 tablespoons butter in a 12-inch pan or skillet over medium-high heat until shimmering. Fry 2 of the chicken breasts until golden-brown on both sides (about 3 to 4 minutes per side). Transfer to warm plate, tent with foil and keep warm. Repeat the same with the remaining 2 chicken breasts.
3. In the same pan with remaining pan grease leftover from the chicken, melt 1 tablespoon of butter. Add the mushrooms and for 2-3 minutes until browned, scraping away at any of the leftover chicken bits off the bottom of the pan.
4. Add the garlic and cook until fragrant, about 1 minute.
5. Pour in the Marsala and the broth and simmer until reduced by half and starting to thicken, (about 10-15 minutes).

6. Pour in the cream and return the chicken back into the sauce. Cook until the sauce thickens (about 3 minutes). Garnish with chopped parsley and serve immediately. (The sauce will continue to thicken off the heat.)

7. Serve over cooked angel hair pasta (or pasta of choice), rice, potatoes, cauliflower rice or zucchini noodles, if desired.

GARLIC HERB BUTTER ROAST CHICKEN

INGREDIENTS

- 4 pound (2kg) whole chicken, at room temperature giblets and neck removed from cavity*
- 1/4 cup unsalted butter, melted
- 3 tablespoons olive oil
- 1/4 cup white wine, (OPTIONAL) -- use a dry wine like a Sauv blanc or Chardonnay
- 1 lemon, halved
- Salt and freshly ground pepper, to taste
- 2 tablespoons fresh chopped parsley
- 4 garlic cloves, minced

- 1 head of garlic roughly peeled and cut in half horizontally through the middle crosswise
- 3 fresh whole rosemary sprigs

INSTRUCTIONS

1. Preheat oven to 430°F | 220°C (400°F or 200°C fan forced). Line a baking tray with foil, or lightly grease a roasting pan.
2. Discard neck from inside the cavity and remove any excess fat and leftover feathers. Pat dry with paper towels.
3. Pour the olive oil, melted butter, wine (if using) and the juice of half a lemon over the chicken, under the skin and inside the cavity. Season chicken liberally on the outside and inside the cavity with salt and pepper. Sprinkle over the parsley.
4. Rub the minced garlic over the chicken, mixing all ingredients together over the chicken and under the skin.
5. Stuff the garlic head into the chicken cavity along with the rosemary sprigs and the squeezed lemon halve. Tie legs together with kitchen string.

6. Place breast-side up into baking tray or roasting pan. Roast for 1 hour and 15-20 minutes, basting half way through cooking time, until juices run clear when chicken thigh is pierced with a skewer.
7. Baste again, then broil for a further 2-3 minutes, until golden.
8. Remove from the oven, cover with foil and allow to stand for 10 minutes before serving. Serve, drizzled with pan juices and remaining lemon half cut into wedges or slices.

ITALIAN HERB BRUSCHETTA CHICKEN

INGREDIENTS

For The Chicken:

- 2 large boneless, skinless chicken breasts halved horizontally to make 4 fillets
- 3 teaspoons Italian seasoning*
- 2 teaspoons minced garlic
- salt to taste
- 1 tablespoon of olive oil (for cooking)

For The Topping:

- 4 Roma tomatoes finely chopped
- 1/4 of a red onion finely chopped (or 3 cloves finely chopped garlic)
- 4 tablespoons shredded fresh basil
- 2 tablespoons olive oil
- salt to taste
- ½ cup freshly shaved parmesan cheese

Balsamic Glaz

- 1/2 cup balsamic vinegar
- 2 teaspoons brown sugar

INSTRUCTIONS

1. Season chicken with Italian seasoning, garlic and salt. Heat oil in a grill pan or skillet, and sear chicken breasts over medium-high heat until browned on both sides and cooked through (about 6 minutes each side). Remove from pan; set aside and allow to rest.
2. Combine the tomatoes, red onion, basil, olive oil in a bowl. Season with salt. Top

each chicken breast with the tomato mixture and parmesan cheese.

3. Serve immediately with balsamic glaze (optional).

For The Balsamic Glaze:

1. (If making from scratch, prepare while chicken is cooking.) Combine sugar (if using) and vinegar in a small saucepan over high heat and bring to the boil. Reduce heat to low; allow to simmer for 5-8 minutes or until mixture has thickened and reduced to a glaze. (If not using sugar, allow to reduce for 12-15 minutes on low heat).

LOADED CAULIFLOWER (LOW CARB, KETO)

INGREDIENTS

- 1 pound cauliflower
- 4 ounces sour cream
- 1 cup grated cheddar cheese
- 2 slices bacon cooked and crumbled
- 2 tablespoons chives snipped
- 3 tablespoons butter

- 1/4 teaspoon garlic powder
- salt and pepper to taste

INSTRUCTIONS

1. Cut the cauliflower into florettes and add them to a microwave safe bowl. Add 2 tablespoons of water and cover with cling film. Microwave for 5-8 minutes, depending on your microwave, until completely cooked and tender. Drain the excess water and let sit uncovered for a minute or two. (Alternately, steam your cauliflower the conventional way. You may need to squeeze a little water out of the cauliflower after cooking.)

2. Add the cauliflower to a food processor and process until fluffy. Add the butter, garlic powder, and sour cream and process until it resembles the consistency of mashes potatoes. Remove the mashed cauliflower to a bowl and add most of the chives, saving some to add to the top later. Add half of the cheddar cheese and mix by hand. Season with salt and pepper.

3. Top the loaded cauliflower with the remaining cheese, remaining chives and

bacon. Put back into the microwave to melt the cheese or place the cauliflower under the broiler for a few minutes.

SPICY BUFFALO CAULIFLOWER BITES PRINT

INGREDIENTS

- 1 head of cauliflower, chopped
- ½ cup whole wheat or gluten-free flour
- ½ cup hot sauce
- 1 tbsp butter or Earth Balance dairy-free butter, melted
- ½ cup water
- Sea salt and garlic powder, to taste

INSTRUCTIONS

1. Preheat oven to 425°F.
2. Chop cauliflower head into 2-3 inch chunks.
3. Mix flour, sea salt, garlic powder and water together in a large bowl.
4. Toss cauliflower chunks in the flour mix, making sure all chunks are coated.
5. Place cauliflower on a baking sheet and roast in the oven for 15-20 minutes.

6. In a separate bowl, melt the butter, then stir together with hot sauce.

7. Remove cauliflower from oven and coat all pieces in hot sauce.

8. Place cauliflower back in the oven and roast for an additional 20-25 minutes.

9. Serve with a side of your favorite blue cheese or ranch dressing.

BUFFALO CHICKEN CASSEROLE

INGREDIENTS

- 1 head cauliflower, cut into florets
- 2 tbsp. extra-virgin olive oil
- Kosher salt
- Freshly ground black pepper
- 12 oz. cream cheese, softened
- 1/3 c. buffalo sauce
- 1/4 c. ranch dressing, plus more for drizzling
- 1/3 c. sliced green onions, plus more for garnish
- 1 tbsp. garlic powder
- 2 c. shredded rotisserie chicken
- 1/2 c. shredded cheddar
- 1/2 c. shredded gouda

INSTRUCTIONS

1. Preheat oven to 450°. In a baking dish, toss cauliflower florets with olive oil and season with salt and pepper.
2. Bake until tender, 20 minutes. Reduce oven temperature to 350°.
3. Meanwhile, in a medium bowl, stir together cream cheese, buffalo sauce, ranch, green onions, and garlic powder until combined. Set aside.
4. Toss rotisserie chicken with roasted cauliflower in baking dish and spread cream cheese mixture on top.
5. Top with cheddar and gouda and bake until cheese is completely melted and bubbly, 20 minutes.
6. Let cool 10 minutes, then drizzle with ranch and garnish with green onions or chives and serve.

BACON WRAPPED GRILLED PEACHES WITH BALSAMIC GLAZE

INGREDIENTS

- 4 large peaches
- 12 ounces bacon
- 60 large basil leaves, plus more for garnish
- extra-virgin olive oil
- balsamic glaze , (store-bought or homemade)

INSTRUCTIONS

1. Set a grill to low heat and preheat for 10 minutes or so, brush the grill grates with a paper towel dabbed in oil. I use grapeseed oil.
2. Wash and dry peaches. Cut each peach in half and then each half into 4 quarters. Place one large basil leaf on each side of the peaches. Cut the bacon slices in half. Wrap each peach slice and basil leaves with a slice of bacon. Pin the loose end of the bacon slice with a toothpick. Repeat with remaining peaches.

3. Brush the bacon wrapped peaches lightly with olive oil so the bacon doesn't stick to the grill. Grill the peaches until the bacon is cooked, turning so all sides are evenly cooked, about 20 minutes.
4. Transfer to a serving platter and remove toothpicks. Drizzle with store-bought or homemade balsamic glaze.
5. Serve hot or at room temperature.

RANCH CAULIFLOWER BITES

INGREDIENTS

- 1 head of cauliflower
- 2 large eggs
- 1 packet ranch seasoning mix
- 1 1/4 shredded sharp cheddar cheese, divided into 1 c and 1/4 c
- 6 strips bacon, cooked and crumbled
- 1 tsp. chives, plus more for topping

INSTRUCTIONS

1. Preheat oven to 375°. Pulse cauliflower in a food processor until it forms large crumbs.
2. Place cauliflower in paper towels or cheesecloth and wring out any excess water. Pour cauliflower crumbles into a large bowl.
3. Add eggs, 1 cup cheese, ranch seasoning, about 3/4s of the bacon, and chives.
4. Grease a muffin tin with cooking spray, then fill each one about 2/3s full. Top with a sprinkle of cheese and crumbled bacon. Bake for about 20 to 22 minutes, or until lightly golden. Garnish with additional chives before serving.

KETO LASAGNA STUFFED PEPPERS

INGREDIENTS

- 1 large red bell pepper
- 1 large green bell pepper
- 1 large yellow bell pepper
- 1 large orange bell pepper
- 2 ½ cups Tomato Meat Sauce
- 1 cup ricotta cheese

- 1 cup mozzarella cheese, shredded
- ½ cup Parmesan cheese, grated
- 1 tablespoon Italian seasoning

INSTRUCTIONS

1. Preheat oven to 400° Line a baking sheet with parchment paper.
2. Slice bell peppers in half lengthwise and remove ribs and seeds. Place pepper halves on baking sheet and bake for 10 minutes on the middle rack.
3. Remove peppers from oven. Fill each pepper with ¼ cup tomato meat sauce.
4. Next, spoon 2 tablespoon of ricotta cheese on top of the meat sauce in each pepper cup. Pour an additional 1 tablespoon meat sauce on top of the ricotta cheese.
5. Top each pepper with 2 tablespoon mozzarella cheese. Bake on middle rack for 12 minutes.
6. Remove peppers from oven. Top each pepper with 1 tablespoon Parmesan cheese and a sprinkle of Italian seasoning. Bake 5 additional minutes on top rack.

ASIAGO CHICKEN WITH BACON CREAM SAUCE

INGREDIENTS

- 1.5 lb chicken breasts (4 small chicken breasts, or 2 large chicken breasts halved)
- 1 ½ tablespoons vegetable oil
- salt and pepper
- 4 garlic cloves minced
- 1 cup chicken stock
- 8 slices bacon , cooked and drained of fat, chopped
- ½ lemon sliced
- 1 cup half and half
- ½ cup asiago cheese shredded
- 2 tablespoons fresh parsley chopped

INSTRUCTIONS

1. Generously season the chicken with salt and pepper on both sides. Heat vegetable oil in a large skillet. Cook chicken breasts on medium-high heat - about 2 minutes on each side, to brown a bit. Chicken doesn't have to

be cooked through - you'll continue cooking it later. Remove the chicken from the skillet.

2. Add minced garlic to the same skillet - cook on medium heat for about 30 seconds, scraping the bottom of the pan. Deglaze the pan with the small amount of chicken stock. Add the remaining chicken stock (total of 1 cup).

3. Add half the bacon (cooked, fat should be drained off, and chopped into small chunks) to the chicken broth.

4. Add the chicken back to the pan, on top of bacon and in the chicken broth. Arrange 5 thin lemon slices around chicken breasts - and cook, simmering on low heat, covered, for about 20 minutes, until the chicken is completely cooked through, and is no longer pink in the center.

5. After the chicken is completely cooked, remove it from the skillet. Remove lemon slices from the skillet - it's very important that you remove them now, do not leave them in for the sauce otherwise it will be too sour. Add 1 cup half and half to the skillet. Bring to boil and mix everything well,

scraping from the bottom. Add ½ cup shredded Asiago cheese and stir to melt completely, about 30 seconds. Immediately reduce to simmer, add chicken breasts back to the skillet and reheat.

6. To serve, spoon some of the sauce over the chicken breasts, and sprinkle with the remaining chopped bacon and chopped parsley.

PALEO MONGOLIAN BEEF (WHOLE30, KETO, GLUTEN-FREE)

INGREDIENTS

Beef Marinade:

- 1 lb skirt steak, beef flap, or sirloin , thinly sliced against the grain
- 2 tbsp coconut aminos
- 1 tbsp Red Boat fish sauce
- 2 tsp toasted sesame oil
- 1 tsp arrowroot starch
- 1/2 tsp baking soda
- 3-4 tbsp avocado or olive oil

Aromatics:

- 3 large cloves garlic, , finely minced
- 3-inch length thinly sliced ginger, , from index through ring finger quantity
- 2 whole red chili peppers (fresno or serrano), , remove seeds, slice to thin strips
- 3 bulbs scallions, , cut into 3-inch length. Separate white and green parts.

INSTRUCTIONS

1. Thin slice beef against the grain. Add ingredients from coconut aminos to baking soda. Mix well and set aside in the fridge.
2. In the meantime, prepare garlic, ginger, scallions, separate white and green parts, and remove the chili pepper seeds and slice them to thin strips
3. In a well-heated stainless steel skillet or cast iron, add 2 tbsp cooking fat. Pan fry the beef in one layer without disturbing over medium-high heat until crisp brown, about 2 minutes then quickly sear the flip side, about 30 seconds. Set the beef and the pan juice aside.

4. Start the skillet dry and add 1 more tbsp cooking oil, saute aromatics with a pinch of salt until fragrant, about 1 minute.
5. Add beef back to the skillet and green scallion parts. Quickly toss to coat the flavor for another 30 seconds. Serve hot and immediately.

ONE PAN PESTO CHICKEN RECIPE

INGREDIENTS

- 2 tablespoons olive oil
- 3 skinless, boneless chicken breasts, cut into 2-inch pieces
- 1 medium red pepper deseeded and sliced
- 5 medium zucchini cut into ribbons or spirals
- 1 pint grape tomatoes halved
- 1/4 cup pesto homemade or store-bought
- mozzarella cheese optional

INSTRUCTIONS

1. Set large pan over medium heat. Drizzle in olive oil. Once the olive oil begins to shimmer, add the chicken pieces and the red

pepper and cook, stirring frequently, until the chicken is cooked throughout, about 8 to 10 minutes. Stir in zucchini, tomatoes, pesto, and mozzarella cheese, if using. Serve immediately.

PINEAPPLE ANGEL FOOD CAKE

INGREDIENTS

- 1 box (1-step) angel food cake mix (I used Betty Crocker)
- 1 large can (about 20 ounces) crushed pineapple, undrained

INSTRUCTIONS

1. Preheat oven to 350F degrees.
2. In a large bowl, stir together the dry cake and the entire can of crushed pineapple with its juice. Stir well until all the dry mix is incorporated. (The mixture will get really foamy.)
3. Pour the batter into a 9x13 pan which has been lightly greased with nonstick cooking spray.

4. Bake at 350F degrees for time specified on the box for size pan. When the sides pull away from pan and toothpick inserted in the center comes out clean, the cake is done. This should take somewhere between 30 and 40 minutes.

5. Remove from the oven and place on a wire rack to cool.